Revitalize with Rest

A Complete and Essential Sleep Wellness Handbook

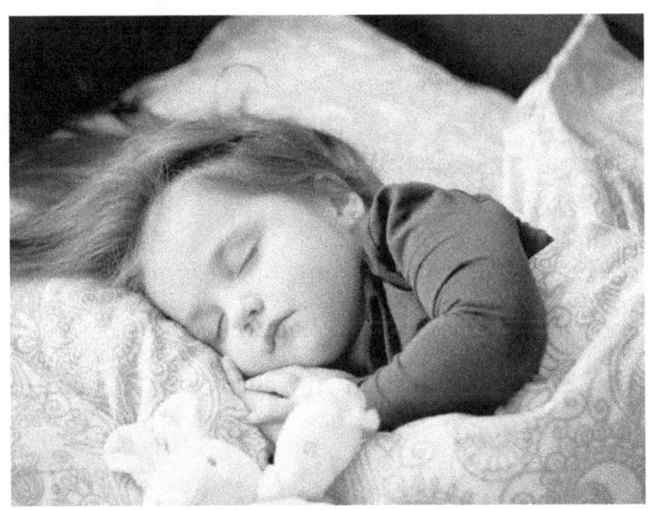

Healthy Happy Me

TABLE OF CONTENTS

Part I: Understanding Sleep Wellness

1.0 Introduction

Dave's eyes felt heavy as he sat at his cluttered desk, struggling to keep his focus on the computer screen. He had been burning the midnight oil for days, working tirelessly to meet an important deadline. Sleep had become a distant memory, replaced by caffeine-fueled nights and restless days.

But Dave was about to learn a valuable lesson—one that would forever change the way he approached his well-being. Little did he know that the key to rejuvenation and peak performance lay not in endless work but in something as simple as a good night's sleep.

1.1 The Importance of Sleep

Sleep, often taken for granted in our fast-paced and productivity-focused world, is a fundamental aspect of human life. It is a natural process that allows the body and mind to rest, repair, and recharge for the challenges of the day ahead. Just like a smartphone that needs to be charged to function optimally, our bodies and brains require sufficient sleep to perform at their best.

The importance of sleep extends beyond mere physical and mental rejuvenation. Research has shown that sleep plays a vital role in memory consolidation, learning, immune function, emotional regulation, and even weight management. Lack of adequate sleep can lead to a range of negative consequences, including impaired cognitive function, decreased productivity, increased stress, and heightened risk of accidents.

1.2 Understanding Sleep Wellness

Sleep wellness encompasses more than just the number of hours spent in bed. It involves the quality and consistency of sleep, as well as factors that influence our ability to fall and stay asleep. Understanding sleep wellness requires delving into the intricacies of sleep cycles, circadian rhythms, and the impact of lifestyle choices on our sleep patterns.

Dave, like many others, had assumed that sleep was merely a time when the body shut down, a passive state in the grand scheme of life. However, he was about to discover that sleep was an active and dynamic process, essential for maintaining a healthy mind and body.

As we embark on this journey with Dave, we will explore the fascinating world of sleep. We will analyze the science behind sleep cycles and stages, uncover the secrets of circadian rhythms, and learn how sleep architecture influences our overall well-being. Likewise, we will explore the various aspects of sleep wellness, from creating a sleep-friendly environment to adopting bedtime routines that promote restful slumber.

Join Dave as he discovers the transformative power of sleep and learns to prioritize his well-being through a comprehensive understanding of sleep wellness. Through his experiences and newfound knowledge, we will gain valuable insights into how we, too, can revitalize our lives with the remarkable benefits of restful sleep. So, let's embark on this enlightening journey together and open the secrets of a well-rested and revitalized existence.

2.0 The Science of Sleep

Sleep is an important and complex biological process that is necessary to maintain overall health and well-being. It allows the body to rest, recover and consolidate memories, ensuring optimal cognitive function and physical performance. Understanding the science of sleep involves exploring many different aspects, such as sleep cycles and stages, circadian rhythms, and sleep structure.

2.1 Sleep Cycles and Stages

Sleep is not a homogeneous state but a dynamic process that goes through distinct cycles and stages. These cycles are generally divided into two main categories: non-rapid eye movement (NREM) sleep and rapid eye movement (REM) sleep. Each cycle usually lasts about 90 to 120 minutes, and a person can experience multiple cycles throughout the night.

NREM Sleep: NREM sleep is further divided into three stages: N1, N2, and N3.

❖ **N1 (Stage 1):** This is the transitional phase between wakefulness and sleep. It is characterized by light sleep, and during this stage, people may experience muscle twitches or sudden jerks.

❖ **N2 (Stage 2):** In this stage, the body starts to relax further, and brain activity slows down. Sleep spindles and K-complexes, which are brief bursts of brain activity, are common during this stage.

❖ **N3 (Stage 3):** Also known as slow-wave sleep (SWS), this is the deep sleep stage where the brain exhibits very slow delta waves. This stage is crucial for physical restoration and rejuvenation, and it is difficult to wake someone during this stage.

REM Sleep: REM sleep is characterized by rapid eye movements and vivid dreams. This step is essential for emotional regulation, memory consolidation, and cognitive processing. During REM sleep, the brain is very active, similar to the waking state, but voluntary muscle activity is inhibited, preventing us from achieving our dreams.

The sleep cycle usually progresses from N1 to N2 to N3 and then into REM sleep. After REM sleep, the cycle begins again with N1 and this pattern repeats throughout the night.

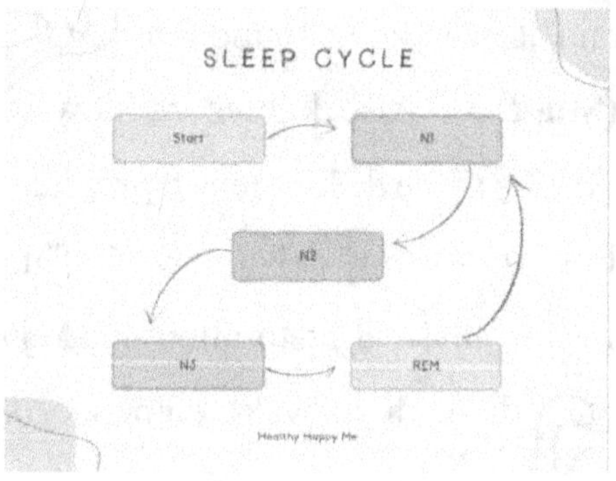

2.2 Circadian Rhythms and Your Body Clock

Circadian rhythms are internal biological clocks that regulate the sleep-wake cycle and various physiological processes in the body. These rhythms are influenced by environmental cues, primarily the light-dark cycle of day and night. The main regulator of the circadian system is the suprachiasmatic nucleus (SCN), a cluster of cells in the hypothalamus.

The circadian rhythm is the internal biological clock that regulates sleep-wake cycles and various physiological processes in the body. These rhythms are influenced by environmental cues, mainly the light-dark cycle of day and night. The major regulator of the circadian system is the suprachiasmatic nucleus (SCN), a group of cells in the hypothalamus.

The SCN receives information about light exposure from the optic nerve in the eye and signals other parts of the brain to release or inhibit hormones, including melatonin, which plays an important role in sleep. Melatonin levels increase in the evening, promoting sleep, and decrease in the morning, helping to wake us up.

Circadian rhythm disturbances, such as time zones or shift work, can lead to sleep disturbances and affect overall health. Establishing a regular sleep schedule, with consistent bedtime and wake-up times, helps keep circadian rhythms working properly and contributes to better quality sleep.

2.3 Sleep Architecture and Brain Activity during Sleep

Sleep architecture refers to the organization and structure of the sleep cycle, including the distribution of sleep stages and their respective durations. Sleep patterns change throughout life and can be influenced by individual factors, such as age, genetics, and lifestyle.

Brain activity during sleep is closely linked to the different stages of sleep. During NREM sleep, the brain gradually decreases its overall activity, with specific regions involved in memory consolidation and physical recovery. In contrast, REM sleep showed increased brain activity, similar to a state of wakefulness. This intense brain activity during REM sleep is thought to be important for emotional processing, learning, and memory.

Various neuroimaging techniques, such as electroencephalography (EEG) and functional magnetic resonance imaging (fMRI), have allowed researchers to better understand brain activity during sleep and its importance to cognitive function and overall health.

Overall, sleep is a multifaceted process involving complex brain cycles, stages, and activities. Understanding the science of sleep can help individuals realize the importance of maintaining healthy sleep patterns and circadian rhythms to support optimal physical and mental health.

Part II : Assessing and Improving Your Sleep Health

3. 0 Assessing Your Sleep Health

Sleep is an essential aspect of overall health, influencing various aspects of physical and mental health. Assessing and improving your sleep health includes understanding your sleep patterns, identifying potential sleep disorders, and taking proactive steps to improve your sleep quality.

Here are some steps you can take to assess and improve your sleep health:

3.1 Identifying Sleep Disorders

Recognizing the presence of a sleep disorder is important for addressing any underlying issues that may be disrupting your sleep. Some common sleep disorders include:

a. Insomnia: Characterized by difficulty falling asleep or staying asleep, waking up too early, or experiencing non-restorative sleep.

b. Sleep Apnea: A condition where breathing repeatedly stops and starts during sleep, leading to disruptions in sleep quality.

c. Restless Legs Syndrome (RLS): An uncomfortable sensation in the legs, usually accompanied by an irresistible urge to move them, which often disrupts sleep.

d. Narcolepsy: A neurological disorder causing excessive daytime sleepiness, sudden sleep attacks, and sometimes cataplexy (sudden loss of muscle tone).

e. Circadian Rhythm Disorders: Conditions where your internal body clock is out of sync with your sleep-wake schedule, such as in shift work sleep disorder or jet lag.

If you think you have a sleep disorder, it is essential to consult a healthcare professional or a sleep specialist. They can help diagnose the problem through a full evaluation, which may include a sleep study or other evaluations.

3.2 Keeping a Sleep Journal

Keeping a sleep journal can provide valuable insights into your sleep patterns and habits. To create a sleep journal, follow these steps:

a. Record Bedtime Routine: Note the activities you engage in before bedtime, such as reading, watching TV, or using electronic devices.

b. Bedtime and Wake Time: Record the time you go to bed and when you wake up each morning.

c. Sleep Duration: Track the total number of hours you sleep each night.

d. Sleep Quality: Rate your sleep quality on a scale from 1 to 10, with 10 being the best.

e. Night-time Awakenings: Note any instances of waking up during the night and the reason for waking up (e.g., bathroom visit, noise, anxiety).

f. Daytime Sleepiness: Rate your daytime sleepiness or fatigue on a scale from 1 to 10, with 10 being extremely sleepy.

g. Stimulants and Alcohol: Keep track of your consumption of stimulants like caffeine and alcohol, as they can impact sleep.

h. Daily Activities: Note any factors that might affect your sleep, such as exercise, stress, or significant life events.

Regularly reviewing your sleep diary can help you identify potential patterns and triggers that affect your sleep. This information can be helpful when discussing your sleep health with a healthcare professional.

3.3 Seeking Professional Help

If you have persistent sleep problems, it is essential to seek professional help. Sleep disturbances can have a significant impact on your physical and mental health, leading to daytime fatigue, decreased productivity, and increased risk of accidents.

A healthcare provider or sleep specialist can perform a thorough evaluation to diagnose any underlying sleep disorders. They may recommend a sleep study where you will be monitored overnight at a sleep center to assess sleep patterns, brain activity, breathing, and other physiological parameters.

Depending on the diagnosis, treatment options may include:

a. Cognitive-Behavioral Therapy for Insomnia (CBT-I): A structured therapeutic approach to address insomnia and promote healthy sleep habits.

b. Continuous Positive Airway Pressure (CPAP) Therapy: For sleep apnea patients, a CPAP machine can help maintain open airways during sleep.

c. Medication: In some cases, sleep medications may be prescribed, but these are typically short-term solutions and are not suitable for long-term use.

d. Lifestyle Changes: A sleep specialist can also recommend lifestyle adjustments, such as improving sleep hygiene, establishing consistent sleep-wake schedules, and managing stress.

Improving your sleep health is a journey that requires patience and a willingness to change. By identifying potential sleep disorders, keeping a sleep diary, and seeking professional help, you can make significant progress in enjoying a restful, rejuvenating sleep that improves your overall quality of life.

4.0 Creating a Sleep-Friendly Environment

Creating a sleep-friendly environment is key to getting a good night's sleep and maintaining overall health. An environment conducive to sleep can significantly improve the quality of our rest. In this section, we'll explore three key aspects of creating a sleep-friendly environment: Optimal Bedroom Setup, Eliminating Sleep Disruptors, and Utilizing Technology for Sleep Improvement.

4.1 Optimal Bedroom Setup

4.1.1 Comfortable bedding:

Start with a comfortable, supportive mattress that matches your sleeping preferences. The right mattress can prevent discomfort and promote better spinal alignment. Pair it with high-quality pillows and soft, breathable bedding to enhance the overall sleeping experience.

4.1.2 Ambient temperature:

Keep the bedroom at a temperature conducive to sleep. The ideal temperature is usually between 60 and 67 degrees Fahrenheit (15 to 20 degrees C). It will be easier for your body to fall asleep and stay asleep in a cool environment.

4.1.3 Lighting:

Invest in curtains or blinds to block any outside light sources, especially if you live in an urban area with street lights or have neighbors with bright outdoor lights. A dark room signals to your body that it's time to rest.

4.1.4 Noise control:

Minimize noise pollution by using earplugs or a white noise machine. White noise can help mask outside sounds and create a more cohesive and calming environment for sleep.

4.1.5 Neat space:

Keep the bedroom neat and organized. A tidy space can reduce feelings of anxiety and promote feelings of calm, making it easier to relax and fall asleep.

4.1.6 Customization:

Decorate your bedroom with soothing colors and relaxing personal items. Avoid stimulating and emotional settings that are potentially stressful or distracting.

4.2 Eliminating Sleep Disruptors

4.2.1 Limit screen time:

Avoid using electronic devices, such as smartphones, tablets, or laptops before bed. The blue light emitted by screens can interfere with the production of melatonin, a hormone responsible for regulating sleep.

4.2.2 Caffeine and Alcohol:

Limit caffeine and alcohol consumption, especially in the hours before bedtime. Both substances can disrupt sleep and reduce sleep quality.

4.2.3 Heavy Meals and Liquid Consumption:

Avoid large meals near bedtime, as they can cause discomfort and disrupt sleep. Also, minimize fluid intake before bed to reduce the likelihood of waking up to go to the bathroom during the night.

4.2.4 Exercises:

While regular exercise can improve sleep quality, intense exercise near bedtime can have the opposite effect. Try to finish the exercise at least a few hours before bedtime.

4.2.5 Pets:

While many people love to sleep with their pets, it's important to consider whether they disrupt your sleep. If your pet's movement or noise bothers you at night, it's best to let them sleep in a separate space.

4.3 Utilizing Technology for Sleep Improvement

Technology can be both a hindrance and an aid as you fall asleep. When used wisely, several technologies can help improve sleep quality. Here are some examples:

1. Sleep monitoring device:

Wearable sleep trackers or smartphone apps can help you track your sleep patterns over time. By analyzing your data, you can identify trends and adjust your sleep habits as needed.

2. Smart lighting:

Consider using a smart light bulb that can simulate a natural sunrise in the morning, gradually increasing the light to wake you up gently. In the evening, these bulbs can emit warmer colors, signaling your body to relax.

3. Relaxing app:

Many apps offer guided meditations, deep breathing exercises, and relaxing sounds to help you wind down before bed.

4. White noise Machine:

White noise can mask disruptive sounds and create a more calming sleeping environment. A white noise generator or app can be especially helpful for light sleepers or those who live in noisy environments.

Remember that while technology can be beneficial, it's essential to establish healthy sleep habits and not just rely on devices for better sleep.

In a nutshell, creating a sleep-friendly environment involves optimizing your bedroom layout, eliminating sleep disturbances, and using technology wisely. By paying attention to these aspects and making the necessary adjustments, you can significantly improve your sleep quality and enjoy better health and overall well-being.

5.0 Developing a Bedtime Routine

A bedtime routine is a set of activities and routines that are done regularly before going to bed. It plays an important role in promoting healthy sleep habits and improving overall sleep quality. In this section, we'll dig deeper into the importance of consistency in your bedtime routine and explore different relaxation techniques and calming activities that can help you get a better night's sleep.

5.1 The Importance of Consistency

Consistency is key when it comes to developing an effective bedtime routine. Our bodies and minds develop out of habit, and following a consistent bedtime ritual signals our internal clock that it's time to relax and prepare to rest. By going to bed and waking up at the same time every day, including weekends, you can regulate your body's sleep-wake cycle, also known as the circadian rhythm.

Consistency in your bedtime routine helps train your brain to associate specific activities with preparation for sleep. Over time, this combination will trigger a natural response in your body, making it easier to fall asleep and sleep soundly through the night. Try creating a bedtime routine that lasts about 30 minutes to an hour, giving yourself plenty of time to relax and blow off steam before trying to go to sleep.

5.2 Relaxation Techniques Before Sleep

Incorporating relaxation techniques into your bedtime routine can be very beneficial in calming the mind, and reducing stress and anxiety, both of which can interfere with falling asleep. Here are some effective relaxation techniques you can try:

a. Deep Breathing: Practice deep, slow breathing to calm your nervous system. Inhale deeply through your nose for a count of 4, hold your breath for 4 counts, and then exhale slowly through your mouth for another count of 4. Repeat this cycle several times.

b. Progressive Muscle Relaxation: Tense and relax each muscle group in your body, starting from your toes and working your way up to your head. This technique helps release physical tension and promotes relaxation.

c. Meditation: Engage in a short meditation session before bed. Focus on your breath, a calming word, or a mental image to clear your mind and prepare for sleep.

d. Visualization: Imagine a peaceful and serene place, such as a beach or a lush forest. Visualize yourself there, engaging your senses to create a vivid and calming mental experience.

e. Aromatherapy: Use essential oils like lavender, chamomile, or bergamot, known for their calming properties. You can diffuse these oils in your bedroom or add a few drops to a warm bath.

5.3 Calming Activities for Better Sleep

Engaging in soothing activities before bed can help you reduce stress and promote relaxation. Here are some activities to consider incorporating into your bedtime routine:

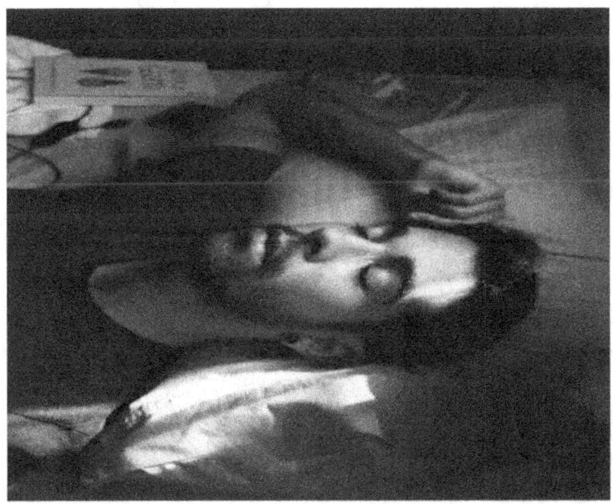

a. Reading: Read a book (preferably in print form rather than electronic) to take your mind off daily worries and immerse yourself in a different world.

b. Gentle Stretching or Yoga: Perform gentle stretching or practice a few calming yoga poses to release tension from your body.

c. Warm Bath: Taking a warm bath can soothe your muscles and promote a sense of relaxation.

d. Journaling: Write down your thoughts, feelings, or any concerns in a journal to unload your mind before sleep.

e. Listening to Calming Music: Listen to soft and soothing music or nature sounds to create a peaceful ambiance in your bedroom.

Remember that the effectiveness of your bedtime routine depends on your consistent commitment. Give yourself time to adjust to your new routine and be patient as you develop healthier sleep habits. Prioritize your sleep as an essential part of your overall health, and you'll likely notice dramatic improvements in sleep quality and energy levels during the day.

Part III: Sleep and Your Lifestyle

6.0 Nutrition and Sleep

Nutrition can have a significant impact on sleep, and certain food choices may promote better sleep quality or disrupt sleep. In this section, we'll explore the relationship between diet and sleep and find out which foods can improve or hinder sleep.

6.1 The Impact of Diet on Sleep Quality

The foods we eat can have a direct effect on the quality of our sleep. Certain nutrients and compounds in foods can affect sleep-wake cycles, brain activity, and hormone regulation, all of which play a role in the length and depth of sleep.

One of the main factors affecting sleep is the neurotransmitter serotonin, which helps regulate mood and sleep. Foods rich in tryptophan, an essential amino acid, can increase serotonin levels in the brain and help improve sleep quality. Tryptophan is a precursor to serotonin, and some foods rich in tryptophan include turkey, chicken, nuts, seeds, soy products, and dairy products. On the other hand, eating multiple meals close to bedtime can lead to irritability and indigestion, making it harder to fall asleep. It is recommended to have dinner at least a few hours before bedtime to allow for good digestion.

6.2 Foods That Promote Better Sleep

Several foods contain nutrients and compounds that support better sleep quality. Some of these include:

a. Complex Carbohydrates: Foods like whole grains, oats, quinoa, and sweet potatoes have a moderate impact on blood sugar levels and can help promote better sleep when consumed in moderation.

b. Magnesium-Rich Foods: Magnesium is a mineral that plays a role in relaxation and sleep regulation. Foods high in magnesium, such as leafy green vegetables, nuts, seeds, and whole grains, can aid in improving sleep.

c. Melatonin-Rich Foods: Melatonin is a hormone that regulates the sleep-wake cycle. Foods like tart cherries, kiwi, and tomatoes contain melatonin and can help improve sleep quality.

d. Herbal Teas: Chamomile and valerian root teas have mild sedative properties and are known for their calming effects, making them popular choices for promoting relaxation before bedtime.

e. Fatty Fish: Fatty fish like salmon, mackerel, and trout are rich in omega-3 fatty acids, which have been associated with improved sleep quality.

f. Bananas: Bananas are a good source of potassium and contain tryptophan, making them sleep-friendly fruit.

6.3 Avoiding Sleep-Disruptive Foods and Beverages

Certain foods and beverages can interfere with sleep and should be consumed in moderation or avoided altogether, especially close to bedtime. These include:

a. Caffeinated Beverages: Coffee, tea, energy drinks, and sodas that contain caffeine can interfere with falling asleep and reduce overall sleep quality. It is best to avoid these beverages in the evening.

b. Alcohol: While alcohol might initially make you drowsy, it can disrupt the later stages of sleep, leading to fragmented and less restorative sleep.

c. Spicy and Acidic Foods: Spicy and acidic foods can cause heartburn and indigestion, making it uncomfortable to sleep.

d. High-Fat and Fried Foods: These foods take longer to digest and may cause discomfort, leading to difficulty falling asleep.

e. Excessive Sugar: High-sugar foods and drinks can cause fluctuations in blood sugar levels, potentially affecting sleep patterns.

f. Excessive Fluids: Consuming too many liquids, especially close to bedtime, may lead to frequent awakenings during the night to use the restroom.

In summary, the impact of diet on sleep quality is significant. Careful food choices including foods that promote better sleep, such as those rich in tryptophan, magnesium, and melatonin, can have a positive effect on sleep. In addition, avoiding or limiting foods and beverages that disrupt sleep can lead to more restful and rejuvenating sleep, which contributes to overall health and well-being. As with any dietary change, it is essential to listen to your body and make the adjustments that best suit your needs and lifestyle.

7.0 Exercise and Sleep

Physical activity and sleep are two essential components of a healthy lifestyle. Engaging in regular physical activity can have a significant impact on the quality and duration of sleep while getting enough sleep is paramount for optimal physical performance and recovery. This section explores the link between exercise and sleep, the best exercises for better sleep, and the optimal timing of exercise to maximize the benefits of sleep.

7.1 The Connection Between Physical Activity and Sleep

The relationship between physical activity and sleep is bidirectional. Regular exercise can promote better sleep quality and duration while getting enough sleep improves athletic performance and aids recovery after exercise. Several mechanisms contribute to this connection:

a) Reduction of Stress and Anxiety: Exercise has been shown to reduce stress and anxiety levels. By engaging in physical activity, the body releases endorphins, also known as "feel-good" hormones, which can help combat stress. Lower stress levels can lead to improved sleep as individuals find it easier to relax and fall asleep.

b) Regulation of Circadian Rhythms: Circadian rhythms are the internal biological processes that regulate the sleep-wake cycle. Physical activity, especially when done outdoors, can help synchronize these rhythms with natural daylight patterns, leading to a more regular sleep schedule.

c) Body Temperature Regulation: Exercise increases core body temperature, and as the body cools down after the workout, it can trigger a natural drop in temperature that promotes sleepiness. However, it is essential to allow enough time for the body to cool down before bedtime, as exercising too close to bedtime may have the opposite effect.

d) Energy Expenditure: Regular exercise helps to expend energy, making the body more physically tired. This physical fatigue, when combined with mental relaxation after exercise, can lead to improved sleep quality.

7.2 Best Exercises for Better Sleep

While any form of physical activity is beneficial for overall health, certain exercises are particularly effective in promoting better sleep:

a) Aerobic Exercises: Activities such as walking, jogging, cycling, swimming, and dancing are excellent choices for improving sleep quality. Aerobic exercises increase heart rate and oxygen consumption, promoting better blood circulation and overall cardiovascular health, which can positively impact sleep.

b) Yoga: Yoga combines physical movement with mindfulness and deep breathing, making it an ideal exercise for improving sleep. The relaxation and stretching techniques in yoga can help reduce stress and promote a sense of calmness before bedtime.

c) Strength Training: Resistance exercises, such as weightlifting or bodyweight exercises like push-ups and squats, can also contribute to better sleep. Strength training helps build muscle, and the body's repair and recovery processes during sleep are essential for muscle growth and repair.

d) Tai Chi: Tai Chi is a low-impact exercise that focuses on slow, deliberate movements and deep breathing. This meditative exercise has been associated with improved sleep quality and relaxation.

7.3 Timing Exercise for Optimal Sleep Benefits

While exercise is generally beneficial for sleep, the timing of your workouts can impact how it affects your sleep:

a) Morning or Afternoon Exercise: For most people, exercising in the morning or afternoon can have positive effects on sleep. Physical activity during these times can help regulate circadian rhythms and boost energy levels during the day, leading to a natural feeling of tiredness in the evening.

b) Avoid Intense Late Evening Workouts: Vigorous exercise too close to bedtime may stimulate the body and mind, making it challenging to fall asleep. Intense workouts elevate heart rate and adrenaline, which can interfere with the body's ability to wind down for sleep. If you prefer exercising in the evening, opt for gentle activities like stretching or yoga, which promote relaxation.

c) Allow Time for Cooling Down: Regardless of the exercise time, it's essential to allow time for a cool-down period before bedtime. This enables the body temperature to gradually return to normal, signaling to the body that it's time to prepare for sleep.

d) Consistency is Key: Regularity in exercise and sleep schedules is crucial for optimizing their benefits. Aim for consistent bedtimes and wake-up times, as well as a consistent exercise routine, to establish a healthy sleep-wake cycle.

In a nutshell, exercise and sleep are interconnected aspects of overall health. Engaging in regular physical activity, choosing the right exercises, and exercising at the right time can improve sleep quality, better overall health, and better athletic performance. Prioritizing exercise and sleep will contribute to a more balanced and healthy lifestyle.

8.0 Managing Stress and Anxiety

Stress and anxiety are common experiences in today's fast-paced world, and they can have a significant impact on our physical and mental health. However, with the right strategies, we can effectively manage and minimize the negative effects of stress and anxiety. In this section, we'll explore the relationship between stress and sleep, coping strategies to reduce stress, and the role mindfulness and meditation play in improving sleep quality.

8.1 The Relationship between Stress and Sleep

The relationship between stress and sleep is bidirectional; Stress can disrupt sleep and not getting enough sleep can increase stress levels. When we're stressed, the body releases stress hormones like cortisol and adrenaline, which can lead to restlessness and difficulty falling asleep. In addition, our minds can race with worries and concerns, making it difficult for us to achieve the peaceful state that leads to sleep.

On the other hand, not getting enough sleep can make us more susceptible to stress. Sleep is essential for the body's recovery and mental processing of emotions and experiences. Without enough good sleep, our ability to cope with stress diminishes and our emotional resilience can suffer.

To break this cycle, it's important to prioritize both stress management and quality sleep.

8.2 Coping Strategies for Reducing Stress

Various coping strategies can help reduce stress levels:

a. Time Management: Organize your schedule and set priorities. This can prevent feeling overwhelmed and reduce the potential for stress to build up.

b. Physical Activity: Regular exercise, such as walking, jogging, or yoga, can release endorphins, which are natural mood lifters and stress reducers.

c. Deep Breathing: Practice deep breathing exercises to activate the body's relaxation response and calm the mind during stressful situations.

d. Social Support: Talk to friends, family, or a therapist about your stressors. Sharing your feelings can provide emotional support and different perspectives.

e. Limit Stimulants: Minimize caffeine and alcohol consumption, especially close to bedtime, as they can interfere with sleep patterns.

f. Hobbies and Relaxation: Engage in activities you enjoy, whether it's reading, painting, or listening to music. These can be effective in reducing stress.

g. Cognitive Reframing: Challenge negative thought patterns and replace them with more positive and constructive ones.

h. Seek Professional Help: If stress becomes overwhelming and unmanageable, consider seeking support from a mental health professional.

8.3 Mindfulness and Meditation for Improved Sleep

Mindfulness and meditation practices can significantly improve sleep quality and reduce stress and anxiety. Mindfulness involves staying present and aware of your thoughts and emotions without judgment. It can be practiced through meditation or simply by being fully engaged in the present moment.

Mindfulness-Based Stress Reduction (MBSR) programs, which often include meditation techniques, are effective in reducing stress and improving sleep in various studies. Here are some mindfulness and meditation techniques that can promote better sleep:

a. Body Scan Meditation: Lie down comfortably and focus your attention on different parts of your body, progressively relaxing each area. This practice helps release physical tension, making it easier to fall asleep.

b. Guided Imagery: Visualize a calming and peaceful scene, like a beach or a forest, and immerse yourself in the sensory details. This can help redirect your mind away from stressful thoughts.

c. Breathing Meditation: Sit or lie down, and concentrate on your breath. Observe each inhale and exhale without trying to control or change your breathing pattern. This practice can calm the mind and induce relaxation.

d. Mindfulness Meditation: Sit comfortably and bring your attention to the present moment—observe your thoughts and feelings without judgment, letting them come and go like passing clouds.

By incorporating these mindfulness and meditation practices into your daily routine, especially before bed, you can establish a sense of inner peace, reduce stress, and improve the overall quality of your sleep.

In summary, managing stress and anxiety is essential to maintaining a healthy and balanced life. By understanding the relationship between stress and sleep, implementing coping strategies, and practicing mindfulness, you can effectively reduce stress levels, improve sleep, and promote a more positive outlook on life. Remember that you can ask someone else or a professional for help if you are having trouble managing stress on your own. Prioritize your health and you will gradually build your resilience and emotional strength to meet life's challenges with greater ease.

Part IV: Addressing Sleep Disorders and Challenges

9.0 Sleep Disorders and Solutions

Many people have sleep disorders that disrupt their peaceful sleep. In this section, we'll dive into three common sleep disorders and explore their causes and potential treatments.

9.1 Insomnia: Causes and Treatments

Insomnia is a common sleep disorder characterized by difficulty falling asleep, staying asleep, or experiencing poor sleep despite the ability to do so. There are two types of insomnia: acute (short-term) and chronic (long-term). The causes of insomnia can vary and may include:

1. Stress and Anxiety: Psychological factors such as excessive worrying, stress, and anxiety can disrupt the ability to relax and fall asleep.

2. Poor Sleep Habits: Irregular sleep schedules, excessive napping during the day, or using electronic devices before bedtime can interfere with sleep quality.

3. Medical Conditions: Certain medical conditions, like chronic pain, asthma, or acid reflux, can make it challenging to find a comfortable sleeping position.

4. Medications: Some medications, particularly stimulants and certain antidepressants, may interfere with sleep.

5. Environmental Factors: Noise, light, or an uncomfortable sleep environment can disturb sleep.

Treatments for insomnia can involve both non-pharmacological and pharmacological approaches:

Non-pharmacological solutions:

- ❖ Cognitive Behavioral Therapy for Insomnia (CBT-I): This structured therapy addresses negative thought patterns and behaviors that contribute to insomnia.

❖ Sleep Hygiene: Implementing healthy sleep habits like maintaining a consistent sleep schedule, creating a relaxing bedtime routine, and limiting caffeine intake can improve sleep quality.

Pharmacological solutions:

❖ Short-term use of sleep aids: In some cases, doctors may prescribe medication to help initiate sleep, but they are usually recommended for short-term use to avoid dependency.

9.2 Sleep Apnea: Diagnosis and Management

Sleep apnea is a sleep disorder characterized by repeated stopping of breathing during sleep, resulting in disrupted sleep cycles. There are three main types of sleep apnea: congested, central, and complex (a combination of congested and central). The most common type is obstructive sleep apnea (OSA), which occurs when the muscles at the back of the throat are unable to keep the airway open.

Diagnosis:

- **Polysomnography:** A sleep study conducted in a sleep center that monitors various physiological parameters during sleep, including brain activity, eye movement, muscle activity, heart rate, respiratory effort, airflow, and blood oxygen levels.

Management:

- Continuous Positive Airway Pressure (CPAP): This is the most common and effective treatment for OSA. A CPAP machine delivers a constant flow of air through a mask, keeping the airway open during sleep.
- Bi-level Positive Airway Pressure (BiPAP): Similar to CPAP but provides different air pressure levels for inhaling and exhaling, which may be more comfortable for some individuals.
- Lifestyle Changes: Weight loss, avoiding alcohol and sedatives before bedtime, and sleeping on one's side can help manage mild cases of sleep

apnea.

9.3 Restless Legs Syndrome: Finding Relief

Restless Legs Syndrome (RLS) is a neurological disorder characterized by an irresistible urge to move the legs, often accompanied by uncomfortable sensations such as crawling, tingling, or burning. These symptoms typically worsen in the evening or at night, leading to difficulties falling asleep.

Causes:

- RLS may have a genetic component and is often associated with conditions like iron deficiency, peripheral neuropathy, and certain chronic diseases.

Finding Relief:

- Medications: Dopaminergic agents, anticonvulsants, and opioids can be prescribed to reduce symptoms in severe cases.

- Iron Supplements: If RLS is linked to iron deficiency, iron supplementation may help alleviate symptoms.
- Lifestyle Changes: Regular exercise, avoiding caffeine and alcohol, and establishing a relaxing bedtime routine can be beneficial.
- Warm Baths and Massages: These techniques can help relax the legs and ease discomfort before bedtime.

It is important to remember that each individual can have a different sleep disorder and the most appropriate treatments should be discussed with a medical professional based on the specific symptoms and medical history of the individual affected.

10.0 Sleep for Different Life Stages

Sleep is a fundamental aspect of human life, and it plays a crucial role in physical, cognitive, and emotional development at different stages of life. The amount of sleep needed and the sleep patterns vary significantly across various age groups. Here, we will explore sleep in three different life stages: Infants and Children, Teenagers and Adolescents, and Older Adults.

10.1 Sleep in Infants and Children

During the early stages of life, sleep is vital for the rapid growth and development of infants and children. Newborns often sleep for around 16 to 20 hours a day, but their sleep is fragmented into short intervals due to their small stomachs needing frequent feeding. As they grow, their sleep patterns become more organized. By the age of 3 to 6 months, most infants start to sleep for longer periods at night.

Infants tend to have irregular sleep-wake cycles, with a greater portion of deep sleep (rapid eye movement - REM sleep). REM sleep is crucial for brain development and processing new information. As they approach one year of age, their sleep patterns gradually resemble those of adults, with a balance of non-REM (NREM) and REM sleep.

Establishing a consistent sleep routine is essential for children's overall health and well-being. This includes regular bedtimes and creating a sleep-conducive environment. Adequate sleep in early childhood fosters learning, memory consolidation, and emotional regulation, and supports physical growth.

10.2 Sleep in Teenagers and Adolescents

During adolescence, there is a shift in sleep patterns due to hormonal changes, social factors, and increased academic demands. Teenagers' circadian rhythm (the internal body clock) tends to shift later, leading to a preference for staying up late and waking up later in the morning. This phenomenon is often referred to as the "delayed sleep phase," and it can result in insufficient sleep, especially on school nights.

The recommended amount of sleep for teenagers is around 8 to 10 hours per night. However, due to early school start times and extracurricular activities, many teenagers experience sleep deprivation. This can have various consequences, including impaired cognitive function, mood swings, reduced academic performance, and an increased risk of accidents.

To promote healthy sleep in teenagers, it is crucial to educate them about the importance of sleep and encourage the establishment of consistent sleep-wake schedules, even on weekends. Limiting screen time before bedtime and creating a relaxing pre-sleep routine can also aid in improving the quality of their sleep.

10.3 Sleep for Older Adults

As people age, their sleep patterns tend to change. Older adults may find it difficult to fall asleep and toss and turn during the night. They tend to wake up more often and may spend less time in deep sleep. In addition, their circadian rhythms may increase, causing them to feel sleepy earlier in the evening and wake up earlier in the morning.

Although there are individual variations, older adults typically need about 7-8 hours of sleep per night. Unfortunately, factors such as medical conditions, medication side effects, and lifestyle changes can disrupt their sleep.

To improve sleep quality in the elderly, maintaining a regular sleep schedule, engaging in regular physical activity, and managing stress are all beneficial. Creating a comfortable sleep environment and limiting caffeine and alcohol consumption near bedtime can also promote better sleep.

In summary, sleep needs and habits vary considerably at different stages of life. Adequate and sound sleep is essential for the overall health, growth, and development of individuals of all ages. By understanding the unique sleep needs of each life stage and implementing healthy sleep habits, individuals can optimize their sleep and enjoy numerous physical and cognitive benefits throughout life.

Part V: Sleep in Specific Situations

11.0 Napping: The Art of Power Naps

Napping, the act of taking a short break during the day, has been practiced by many cultures for centuries. In recent times, the scientific community has recognized the many benefits of napping, which has led to a growing interest in the art of energizing naps. Power naps are short, focused naps designed to increase productivity, improve cognitive function, and improve overall health. Here, we'll explore the benefits of napping and provide tips on how to nap effectively.

11.1 The Benefits of Napping

1. Increased Alertness: A well-timed nap can combat drowsiness and help you feel more alert and attentive. It's particularly useful for combating that mid-afternoon slump that many people experience.

2. Enhanced Cognitive Function: Napping can lead to improved memory, creativity, and problem-solving skills.

During sleep, the brain consolidates information and forms new connections, enhancing cognitive abilities.

3. Stress Reduction: Napping can help reduce stress and promote relaxation. A short nap can give your body and mind a break, allowing you to better cope with daily stressors.

4. Improved Mood: Napping can have positive effects on mood, reducing feelings of irritability and enhancing emotional stability.

5. Boosted Physical Performance: Athletes often use napping as a tool to enhance physical performance and promote muscle recovery.

6. Heart Health: Regular napping has been associated with a reduced risk of heart disease and lower blood pressure.

7. Enhanced Learning: Napping after learning something new can aid memory retention and information processing.

8. Increased Productivity: Taking a short nap can refresh your mind and increase productivity, making you more efficient in your tasks.

11.2 How to Nap Effectively

While napping can offer numerous benefits, not all naps are created equal. To reap the advantages of power napping, follow these tips:

1. Keep It Short: Power naps are typically 10 to 30 minutes long. Longer naps may lead to sleep inertia, causing grogginess upon waking.

2. Find the Right Time: Aim to nap during the early afternoon when your energy levels tend to dip. Napping too close to bedtime may interfere with night-time sleep.

3. Create a Relaxing Environment: Find a quiet, dimly lit space with a comfortable place to lie down. Use a blanket or eye mask to block out light and noise.

4. Set an Alarm: To avoid oversleeping, set an alarm for the desired nap duration. This will prevent you from slipping into a deep sleep cycle.

5. Practice Consistency: If possible, try to nap at the same time each day. Consistency can help your body adapt to the routine and optimize the benefits of napping.

6. Limit Caffeine and Heavy Meals: Consuming caffeine or heavy meals close to nap time can make it harder to fall asleep. Opt for a light snack if needed.

7. Don't Feel Guilty: Napping is a healthy way to recharge, so don't feel guilty about taking a short break during the day.

8. Avoid Screens: Before napping, avoid electronic devices such as phones, tablets, and computers. The blue light emitted by screens can disrupt your sleep-wake cycle.

Remember that a nap is no substitute for a regular and quality night's sleep. It should complement your usual sleep routine, not replace it. If you feel excessively tired during the day despite taking a nap, you should discuss your sleep habits with a healthcare professional to rule out any sleep disorders or underlying health conditions.

12.0 Travel and Jet Lag

Traveling can be an enjoyable experience, whether for business or pleasure. However, crossing time zones often leads to time zone drift, a temporary sleep disorder that affects our internal body clocks. The time zone difference occurs because our circadian rhythm, the internal biological clock that regulates our sleep-wake cycles, is out of sync with the new time zone. This can lead to feelings of fatigue, trouble sleeping on time, irritability, and difficulty concentrating. To get the most out of your trip and minimize the effects of jet lag, here are a few tips to consider:

12.1 Minimizing Jet Lag Effects

1. Gradually Adjust Sleep Schedule: If possible, start adjusting your sleep schedule a few days before you leave. If you're traveling east, try to go to bed and wake up an hour earlier each day. For the westward journey, do the

opposite, going to bed and waking up an hour later each day. This gradual change can help your body adapt to the new time zone.

2. Choose Flights Wisely: Consider your flight schedule when booking. If you're traveling east, try to catch your flight arriving in the evening, so you can get some sleep as soon as you arrive. If you're heading west, choose a morning or daytime flight to keep you awake for the day.

3. Stay Hydrated: Dehydration can make jet lag symptoms worse. Drink plenty of water before, during, and after your flight. Avoid excessive caffeine and alcohol, as they can dehydrate you and disrupt your sleep.

4. Get Sunlight Exposure: Natural light is a powerful regulator of our circadian rhythms. Spend time outdoors in the sun, especially in the morning, as this can help your body adapt to the new time zone more quickly.

5. Short Naps: While you may want to take a long nap after a tiring flight, it's best to take a short (20-30 minute)

nap during the day to avoid interfering with your ability to sleep at night.

6. Melatonin Supplements: Some travelers find melatonin supplements helpful in adjusting to a new time zone. Consult a healthcare professional before using them as they may not be suitable for everyone and may interact with certain medications.

7. Be Patient: Give your body time to adjust. Jet lag is a temporary condition that usually resolves on its own within a few days. Avoid stressing about it, as anxiety can worsen sleep problems.

12.2 Sleep Tips for Frequent Travelers

1. Create a Sleep-Friendly Environment: Whether you stay in a hotel, Airbnb, or other accommodation, try to create a comfortable sleeping environment. Use blackout curtains, earplugs, and white noise machines to minimize distractions.

2. Stick to a Sleep Routine: If possible, maintain a consistent sleep schedule, even during your travels. Going

to bed and waking up at the same time each day can help regulate your circadian clock.

3. Limit Screen Time Before Bed: The blue light emitted by electronic devices can interfere with your ability to fall asleep. Avoid screens at least an hour before bed to improve sleep quality.

4. Use Relaxation Techniques: If you're having trouble falling asleep in your new surroundings, try relaxation techniques like deep breathing, meditation, or gentle stretching to help you relax before bed.

5. Avoid Heavy Meals and Stimulants: Large, heavy meals and stimulants like caffeine close to bedtime can disrupt your sleep. Opt for light, easily digestible dinners and avoid caffeine in the evening.

6. Stay Active: Engage in regular physical activity during your travels. Exercise can promote better sleep and help reduce stress.

7. Stay Consistent with Sleep Aids: If you use sleeping pills at home, consider taking them with you when you travel. Maintaining a consistent sleep routine, including

sleeping pills if prescribed by your doctor, can be beneficial.

Remember that everyone's body is different and what works for one person may not work for another. Experiment with these tips to find a routine that works best for you. By taking steps to minimize the effects of jet lag and adopting healthy sleep habits, you can make your travel experience more enjoyable and relaxing.

13.0 Shift Work and Sleep

Shift work refers to any work schedule that falls outside of regular "9 to 5" working hours. Many industries, such as healthcare, transportation, manufacturing, and hospitality, require employees to work non-traditional hours, which can significantly affect their sleep and overall health. The vagaries of shift work can lead to disruptions in circadian rhythms, making it difficult for shift workers to get enough sound sleep.

13.1 Coping with Irregular Work Schedules

Coping with irregular working hours is crucial for shift workers to maintain good health and productivity. Here are some strategies that can help:

1. Establish a Consistent Sleep Routine: Even with varying hours, try to establish a regular sleep schedule as much as possible. Going to bed and waking up at the same time every day, even on days off, can help regulate your body's internal clock.

2. Create a Relaxing Bedtime Ritual: Engage in calming activities before bed, such as reading a book, taking a warm bath, or practicing relaxation techniques. This can signal to your body that it's time to relax and prepare for bed.

3. Optimize Your Sleep Environment: Make your bedroom sleep-friendly by keeping it cool, dark, and quiet. Consider using blackout curtains, earplugs, or a white noise machine to prevent distractions.

4. Limit Caffeine and Stimulants: Avoid consuming caffeine and other stimulants near bedtime as they can interfere with your ability to fall asleep.

5. Manage Light Exposure: Exposure to bright light, especially blue light from electronic devices, can disrupt your sleep-wake cycle. Limit screen time before bed and consider using a blue light filter on your device.

6. Take Short Naps: If you're feeling too tired, naps (20-30 minutes) during breaks can help reduce sleepiness without affecting nighttime sleep.

7. Communicate with Your Employer: If possible, contact your employer about your preferred work schedule. Some people may find it easier to fit into specific shifts, so discussing your preferences may lead to a more suitable arrangement.

8. Plan for Adequate Rest between Shifts: If possible, make sure you have enough time to rest between shifts. Shorter rest periods can negatively impact your sleep quality and overall health.

13.2 Strategies for Shift Workers to Improve Sleep

Improving the sleep of shift workers requires careful attention to daytime and nighttime sleep habits. Here are some strategies to consider:

1. Gradual Shift Changes: If you rotate shifts, try to request a schedule that allows for gradual rather than abrupt shifts. This gives your body more time to adjust to the new sleep-wake pattern.

2. Use Bright Light Exposure: Exposure to bright light during your waking hours, especially during the night shift, can help regulate your circadian rhythm. Use bright lights at work and wear sunglasses when you get home in the morning to minimize exposure to daylight.

3. Stay Active: Regular exercise can improve sleep quality, reduce stress and improve mood. Build physical activity into your routine, but avoid vigorous exercise too close to bedtime.

4. Healthy Eating Habits: Shift workers should pay attention to their diet. Eat well-balanced meals and avoid heavy, fatty, or spicy foods near bedtime as they can cause discomfort.

5. Limit Caffeine and Alcohol: Caffeine and alcohol can disrupt sleep. While it's best to avoid them near bedtime, if you do consume them, do it in moderation.

6. Nap Strategically: Naps during breaks may help, but avoid long naps or naps too close to bedtime as this can interfere with night-time sleep.

7. Stay Connected: Maintain social relationships with family and friends. A strong support system can help reduce stress and improve overall health.

8. Consider Sleep Aids with Caution: If you have trouble sleeping, consult your doctor before using sleeping pills.

They should be used with caution and only as a short-term solution.

Remember that everyone's sleep needs are different, so it's important to find the strategies that work best for you. Prioritize sleep and take steps to manage the challenges of shift work, as good sleep is important to your overall health, safety, and performance.

Part VI: Enhancing Sleep Naturally

14.0 Enhancing Sleep Quality Naturally

Unfortunately, many people struggle with sleep-related problems such as insomnia, tossing, or difficulty falling asleep. While there are many sleep aids available, some people prefer natural remedies to improve sleep quality. In this section, we'll explore herbal and complementary treatments as well as aromatherapy and essential oils that can naturally help relax and improve sleep.

14.1 Herbal Remedies and Supplements for Sleep

1. Valerian Root: Valerian root is one of the best-known herbal remedies for sleep. It has been used for centuries to promote relaxation and relieve insomnia. Valerian root is thought to increase levels of gamma-aminobutyric acid (GABA) in the brain, a neurotransmitter that helps calm and reduce anxiety.

2. Chamomile: Chamomile is a popular herb known for its soothing properties. It contains apigenin, an antioxidant that binds to certain receptors in the brain, promoting relaxation and sleepiness.

3. Lavender: Lavender is commonly used in aromatherapy, but it can also be taken as a supplement to improve sleep quality. Studies show that lavender can reduce stress and anxiety, which are often causes of sleep disturbances.

4. Passionflower: Passionflower is another herb commonly used to treat sleep disorders. It can increase GABA levels in the brain, leading to a more relaxed state and better sleep.

5. Melatonin: Melatonin is a hormone naturally produced by the body to regulate sleep-wake cycles. It is available as a dietary supplement and may be helpful for people with air sickness or irregular sleep patterns.

6. Magnesium: Magnesium is a mineral that plays an important role in promoting relaxation and calming the nervous system. Some studies suggest that magnesium supplements can improve sleep quality.

It's important to note that while supplements and herbs may work for some people, they may not work for everyone and it's always a good idea to consult a medical professional before starting any new supplement, especially if you're taking other medications or have any underlying health conditions.

14.2 Aromatherapy and Essential Oils for Relaxation

Aromatherapy is the use of essential oils derived from plants to promote relaxation, reduce stress, and improve sleep. The following essential oils are known for their soothing properties:

1. Lavender Oil: Lavender essential oil is one of the most popular oils used for relaxation and sleep. Its soothing aroma can help reduce anxiety and improve overall sleep quality.

2. Roman Chamomile Oil: Roman chamomile has a sweet floral scent that can create a feeling of calm and tranquility. Inhaling its aroma before bed can help you fall asleep faster.

3. Bergamot Oil: Bergamot essential oil has a fresh lemon scent. It is said to reduce stress and promote relaxation, which is beneficial for people with insomnia or sleep disturbances caused by anxiety.

4. Ylang-Ylang Oil: Ylang-ylang has a rich floral scent that can help relieve stress and promote feelings of well-being. It may also help lower blood pressure, which can contribute to a more relaxed state that leads to sleep.

5. Sandalwood Oil: Sandalwood has a woody, earthy scent that can help calm the mind and promote relaxation before bed.

To use essential oils for sleep, you can:

- Add a few drops of your chosen oil to the diffuser in your bedroom before bed.
- Mix a few drops with a carrier oil like coconut oil and apply it to your wrists or neck as a soothing scent.
- Make a pillow spray by mixing water with a few drops of essential oils and lightly spritzing on your pillows and sheets.

It is essential to use pure, high-quality essential oils and do a patch test on your skin to check for any allergic reactions before using them on a larger scale.

In conclusion, combining herbal remedies, supplements, and aromatherapy with essential oils can be a natural and effective way to improve sleep quality and promote relaxation. However, individual responses to these methods can vary, and maintaining consistent sleep habits, maintaining a comfortable sleep environment, and practicing good sleep hygiene is key to achieving the best results. As always, if sleep problems are persistent or severe, it is important to see a medical professional to address any underlying health problems.

15.0 Embracing Technology for Better Sleep

Advancements in technology have paved the way for innovative solutions to improve our sleep patterns and overall sleep quality. Here, we will explore two major ways technology is helping us achieve better sleep: Sleep Tracking Devices and Apps, and Smart Home Solutions for Sleep Enhancement.

15.1 Sleep Tracking Devices and Apps

Sleep monitoring devices and apps are designed to track and analyze various aspects of your sleep patterns, providing valuable insights into your nighttime sleep. These devices typically use sensors and algorithms to collect data including movement, heart rate, breathing patterns, and even environmental factors like noise and light levels. Here's how they contribute to better sleep:

1. Personalized Sleep Analysis: Sleep tracking devices and apps create personalized sleep profiles by collecting data over time. They can identify patterns and disturbances, such as snoring, sleep apnea, or restless leg syndrome, which may be affecting your sleep quality.

2. Sleep Efficiency Metrics: These technologies can calculate your sleep efficiency, which is the percentage of time you spend asleep in bed. By understanding your sleep efficiency, you can adjust your sleep schedule and habits to maximize restorative sleep.

3. Sleep Recommendations: Based on the data collected, sleep-tracking apps can offer personalized recommendations to improve your sleep. This may include suggestions for adjusting your bedtime routine, creating a sleep-conducive environment, or changing your sleep duration.

4. Wake-Up Optimization: Many sleep tracking devices come with smart alarms that wake you up during your lightest sleep phase, minimizing grogginess and helping you feel more refreshed in the morning.

5. Sleep Coaching: Some apps offer sleep coaching features that provide educational content and tips to help you establish healthy sleep habits and address sleep-related issues.

15.2 Smart Home Solutions for Sleep Enhancement

Smart home technology has expanded to include devices and systems specifically designed to improve sleep quality. These solutions often integrate with other smart devices in your home to create a personalized and soothing sleep environment. Here are some examples of how smart home technology can aid in better sleep:

1. **Smart Lighting**: Smart bulbs and lighting systems can be programmed to mimic natural light patterns, gradually dimming as bedtime approaches, and gently brightening in the morning to simulate a sunrise. This helps regulate your circadian rhythm and promotes better sleep-wake cycles.

2. **Temperature Control**: Smart thermostats can maintain an optimal sleep temperature in your bedroom, ensuring it's neither too hot nor too cold, as extreme temperatures can disrupt sleep.

3. **White Noise Machines**: Smart white noise machines can create a consistent and soothing sound environment, masking disruptive noises and helping you fall asleep faster and stay asleep.

4. **Smart Mattresses and Pillows**: Some mattresses and pillows come equipped with sensors to track your sleep movements and provide feedback on your sleeping positions and comfort levels. They may even adjust their firmness or support throughout the night for enhanced comfort.

5. **Integration with Sleep Trackers**: Smart home devices can integrate with sleep tracking apps, allowing for more comprehensive sleep data collection and analysis. This integration helps you make more informed decisions about your sleep environment and habits.

Using technology for better sleep requires a balanced approach. While these tools can be very beneficial, it is essential to remember that good sleep hygiene and healthy sleep habits are still important factors for achieving optimal sleep. Technology can be a supportive ally in the quest for better sleep, but it is essential to use it consciously and in combination with other lifestyle adjustments for long-term improvements in sleep quality.

Part VII: Embracing Rest and Breaks

16.0 The Power of Naps and Rest Breaks

Rest is an essential aspect of maintaining overall health and productivity. Incorporating regular rest and naps into daily life can have many positive effects on physical, mental, and emotional health. In this section, we'll explore the importance of rest and the benefits of incorporating breaks into our daily routines.

16.1 Incorporating Rest into Daily Life

In our fast-paced advanced society, many people tend to disregard the significance of rest, frequently prioritizing work and other commitments over their well-being. In any case, research has consistently shown that taking regular breaks all through the day can essentially enhance efficiency and in general performance. Here are a few practical ways to incorporate rest into everyday life:

1. Short Rest Breaks: Throughout the workday, take short breaks every hour or two. Step away from your desk,

stretch, or simply walk around the office. These brief moments of rest allow your mind to recharge and prevent burnout.

2. Power Naps: A short nap of around 20-30 minutes can work wonders for both cognitive and physical functioning. It helps improve alertness, memory, and mood, making you more focused and productive once you wake up.

3. Lunch Break: Utilize your lunch break wisely by stepping outside, enjoying a balanced meal, and engaging in activities that help you relax and unwind.

4. Mindfulness and Meditation: Incorporate mindfulness practices into your day. Taking a few minutes to meditate or practice deep breathing can help reduce stress and increase mental clarity.

5. Physical Activity: Engage in light physical activities during breaks, such as walking, stretching, or yoga. Exercise boosts endorphin levels and improves overall well-being.

6. Weekend Rest: Make sure to allow yourself time for relaxation and enjoyment during the weekends. Avoid overcommitting to tasks and allow yourself to recharge fully.

16.2 The Benefits of Regular Breaks

The advantages of incorporating regular breaks into your daily routine extend beyond just feeling refreshed. Here are some significant benefits of taking breaks:

1. Improved Focus and Concentration: Breaks prevent mental fatigue, allowing your mind to reset and focus better when you return to tasks.

2. Enhanced Creativity: Rest provides an opportunity for your brain to make new connections and promotes creative thinking.

3. Stress Reduction: Taking breaks helps lower stress levels, preventing the negative impact of chronic stress on your health.

4. Better Memory Consolidation: During rest, your brain processes and consolidates information, leading to better memory retention.

5. Physical Well-being: Regular breaks can reduce the risk of physical ailments associated with prolonged sitting or repetitive tasks.

6. Increased Productivity: Counterintuitive as it may seem, incorporating breaks can improve overall productivity. It prevents burnout and allows you to work efficiently when you are engaged.

7. Emotional Recharge: Breaks provide time to process emotions and reduce feelings of overwhelm.

8. Improved Decision-making: Rested minds are better equipped to make sound decisions and judgments.

9. Better Work-Life Balance: By prioritizing rest, you create a healthier work-life balance, leading to greater overall satisfaction.

In conclusion, taking regular breaks and incorporating naps into your daily routine is not a sign of laziness but rather a strategy to optimize your health and productivity. Rest is an essential part of a healthy lifestyle and by adopting it, you can lead a more balanced and fulfilling life.

Part VIII: Conclusion

17.0 Conclusion: Your Journey to Optimal Sleep Wellness

In this enlightening journey, we followed Dave's transformative experience and learned an invaluable lesson about prioritizing sleep for overall health. As we conclude our exploration of sleep health, let's reflect on the key insights gained and the path to optimal rest and rejuvenation.

- Sleep's Significance:

Dave's story sheds light on the fundamental importance of sleep in our lives. Just like smartphones need to be charged to function optimally, our bodies and minds need enough sleep to function at their best. Sleep is not just a passive state; it's an active process that allows the body to rest, repair and recharge while facilitating memory consolidation, learning, immune function, emotional regulation, and weight control.

- Understanding Sleep Wellness:

Good sleep goes beyond hours in bed. It includes the quality and regularity of sleep, which is influenced by factors such as sleep cycles, circadian rhythms, and lifestyle choices. By delving deeper into the science behind these aspects, we can better understand the profound impact sleep has on our overall health.

- Prioritizing Restful Slumber:

Dave's midnight oil-burning experience has taught us that sleep neglect can lead to negative consequences, including impaired cognitive function, decreased productivity, increased stress, and increased risk of accidents. To prioritize good sleep, we must create an environment conducive to sleep and adopt bedtime routines that promote peaceful sleep.

- Embracing the Transformative Power of Sleep:

As we saw in Dave's Journey, embracing the transformative power of sleep can revitalize our lives. By incorporating sleep health principles into our daily routine, we can unlock the remarkable benefits of rejuvenation, improved cognitive function, improved productivity, and a stronger immune system.

The insights we gain through Dave's experience and our discovery of sleep health allow us to embark on a journey toward optimal health. Remember that a good night's sleep is not a luxury but a necessity, and it holds the key to unlocking our true potential.

As we come to the end of this book, let us understand that sleep is a precious gift we can give ourselves every night. By respecting the need to rest and rejuvenate, we set the stage for a healthier, happy, and more fulfilling life.

May you find the balance and wisdom needed to make good sleep the foundation of your life, and may your path be enlightened by the transforming power of a fully rested and revitalized existence. Sweet dreams await you on your journey to optimal healthy sleep.